BREAK THE ICE
TALK TO STRANGERS
& WIN YOUR FEARS

Discover How To Start The Fire And Make Interesting Conversation, Taking Small Talk To The Next Level

Steve Lowndes & Ian Leil

errors, omissions, or inaccuracies.

errors, omissions, or inaccuracies.

TABLE OF CONTENTS

CHAPTER 1:
HOW DO YOU START A CONVERSATION WITH SOMEONE?

For a variety of reasons, which can be getting to know more new people, trying to build a relationship with someone or just having a good time that night and an enjoyable experience, very often people ask themselves:

"How do I start talking to someone in a bar?"

"How can I talk to that girl at the party?"

"How do I make friends with that person at that event?"

Now, truth be told, yes, there may be specific differences in the way that you will want to talk to these people depending on the scenario.

But, the thing is that most of the time what really happens is that you end up just standing there thinking about all the different possible things you could say without actually taking any action.

When the time comes, when it's time for you to say something, you are blocked by a myriad of thoughts and you don't say anything.

Let's say that you had a general method of approach that you could use on anyone, anywhere, to start a conversation.

It would be great right?

Well then just allow me to show you how it's done.

I will teach you three methods to strike a conversation with anyone that will become so natural to you that they will turn into just a reflex so that you will be able to finally speak up and meet some interesting people.

Without getting lost in chitchat, let's dive straight into it: this is how you can easily and successfully start a conversation with anyone.

CHAPTER 2:
THE MENTAL SEARCH METHOD

The first method we're going to see is used to make a practical change in the way you start a conversation with someone, by affecting your mindset.

We call it "The Mental Search Method": let's see how it has anything to do with conversations and how it will change your mentality.

Why "The Mental Search Method"? You know the way you would search for words or facts on Google? Great, you have to do the same thing but in your head.

Let me explain this a little bit more in depth.

Nowadays whenever you want to know something, you won't ask someone else directly or say it out loud, you will most likely look it up online.

If you want to know the best restaurants in the area, you will check them out on yelp or tripadvisor and so on.

But what if you did actually ask someone else? Isn't that a super easy yet effective way to engage in some small talk?

I remember for example the other day when I was at the gym, there was going to be a big football game that night and as someone new in the area, I had no idea where to watch it. So I just randomly asked a guy and just like that we spoke for a good 10 minutes and I ended up meeting up with him that night at the pub to watch the fight.

So the trick is, ask all those questions that come up in your mind out loud to people around you or directly to the person you want to talk to.

You can practically use this technique with anyone; we advise that you use it with people you don't know at all, to practice your technique and to make sure that you use it more and more naturally.

Obviously to start it is also fine with groups or people you know.

Let's make another example.

I recently moved to Beverly Hills. Nice place. I really like it.

This is what I did to start getting to know people there:

The first question you want to ask to a person or people nearby is: "Do you live here?"

You could say, for example, "What's the reason why you like it so much here?" or "If you had to convince someone who just moved here to stay, what would you tell them to visit?"

In this way, you will be able to not only meet new people or entire groups of people, you will also discover new places, create new relationships, make new friends or even just have a chat with a stranger for a few minutes.

I'll give you another scenario. Imagine that you're walking somewhere and suddenly you hear someone speaking a language you recognize or you even speak yourself (it really doesn't matter if you don't, showing interest and curiosity is more than enough).

You could just ask them, for example, "Hi, where are you from?" "Are you a tourists?" "Are you visiting here?".

You might think that these are stupid and trivial examples, but there is an important lesson in all this, which we will explain more in depths later on:

It doesn't matter how you start a conversation, the truly important thing is how you continue it. Therefore, the first thing you say is of little to no importance (unless you offend the other person, which we wouldn't honestly suggest).

CHAPTER 3:
THE TRUE SECRET TO KEEP THE CONVERSATION GOING

The goal after starting a conversation is to keep it up.

The way you can continue your conversation is what creates a real bond with that new person or group of people.

Here's another little secret for you, what truly matters is to lead the conversation towards the emotional plane, and then ask the other person variations of the question "How do you feel" (right now or about something and/or someone).

So, let's go back to one of the previous examples.

We broke the ice but we will truly only engage in a real conversation from the moment we ask that very important question "how do you feel?".

So we could ask someone "How do you feel about tonight?" "Are you excited about what's happening?" "What do you think about this and that?"

This way you will deepen your bond with your interlocutor and will start creating a connection based on feelings towards something.

"How do you like it here? What's your favorite thing?" when you ask them a feeling question that's when we get to people's sensations and feelings, that's when the real one-on-one game begins and we can keep the conversation interesting, engaging and fluid.

This connects directly to our second method: this is what we will call the twitter method.

If we use google to ask questions, twitter is where we go to make a statement.

I was at a club the other night.

At one point I see a person dressed in a very shiny suit who looked almost like an astronaut.

Basically, I grabbed the person who was standing right next to me and I said, "Hey, you gotta see this one. An astronaut just walked right into the club!"

And that's it, that's really how simple it is, after that we started talking and our conversation started.

Now, the fundamental point of these methods you're discovering is that you should not be going to the person or group of people you're interested in and try to start a conversation with a question or phrase you've already planned before or you have been thinking about for hours.

The problem a lot of people have is that they sit there thinking and thinking, looking for something to say without actually taking any action.

Overthinking never helps in these spontaneous situations.

Many people think they should break the ice with a compliment, and then they just get stuck thinking about what they should even compliment or how to phrase it.

And let's be honest, say that you want to open your conversation by complimenting someone's outfit and they're just wearing a white t shirt and jeans. Chances are your comment will not sound credible or genuine at all.

But when you put aside that fixation for searching at all cost for the right thing to say, which often turns out to be useless effort, and you simply go with the flow of genuine thoughts going through your head, you will always have something to say that no matter how stupid, silly or trivial it may seem at first, will allow you to start talking to someone.

I can't stress this enough, the real focus of the conversation, what really matters, is not what you say at first.

Believe it or not, there are countless people out there who can't wait to have a conversation with someone…

So next time you're out there thinking, "Oh my God, it's so hot today, I'm roasting", just say it out loud. Boom, twitter method.

It's very likely that someone close to you will say something like, "Yes this is unbelievable, it's so hot, isn't it? "

Now you can level the field right away.

You can continue with "It's absurd, isn't it? I don't know if I can take it. I was almost thinking about moving somewhere else, what do you think?"

And that's really it, remember that an emotional response is what you are truly looking for.

When you get to talk about each other's feelings, you're starting to have a real conversation…

CHAPTER 4:
THE THIRD TECHNIQUE

The third method is something very effective in closed social settings and the best part is that it's nothing more than a simple sentence.

Virtually we are talking about any kind of environment really, a club, a bar, your university and so on.

The unconscious expectation of any kind of person or group of people who attend these places is to be social, and therefore to talk to people.

As a result, these are systematically great places to be social with other people.

The method is quite simple: you go over to a person (even in a group) and you tell them: "Hey, I don't think I've met you yet. I'm Fred", while reaching out for a handshake.

It's really that simple.

It's a technique that works almost always and it's great because it communicates unconsciously a number of things about yourself to the other person.

First of all, it shows that you are a sociable person, since you're practically starting the conversation in a very natural way.

Secondly, it makes it clear that people should know each other in these contexts and that it's weird that that person has not gotten to know you yet.

It's like saying, "You know, I don't think I've met you yet, we should have definitely met by now."

As a reflex, people will shake your hand as you reach out to shake theirs, they will follow you and be interested in what you say.

Again, what you'll want to do next is connect to the feelings of the person you're talking to, by asking questions such as, "are you having fun? What do you like about this place? What brings you here tonight? "

This way, you'll start the real conversation and your relationship will deepen creating a superficial bond.

Remember, don't worry too much about how the conversation starts. Just start it and dive straight into it.

We still want to give you more ways to continue your conversations so that you don't have embarrassing moments of silence and you can always have something to say even when you're in trouble, so now we'll cover how to make small talk.

CHAPTER 5:
SMALL TALK

We'll now give you simple and effective methods to use to engage in small talk with anyone, to make your conversations fluid, easy going and fun so that the person you are talking to will like you almost instantly!

What's the point of making small talk?

The function of small talk is to keep a conversation going successfully and to prevent it from getting stuck in a dead end.

The goal of making small talk is still the same as doing conversation: to check if you can get along with a person, to see if you can have a relationship of sort with that person, or to see if you like that person or not. As a result, you can create friendships, deeper bonds and romantic relationships.

Without getting lost in chitchat, we will immediately see some simple and effective ways to make small talk and to be liked straight away by the people we talk to.

CHAPTER 6:
SURPRISE THEM

The first method, that usually surprises most people, is to go for a compliment plus a cold-read of the person you are talking to.

The other day I was chatting with a group of people I had just met. I made a joke and a girl just naturally said "Oh you're so funny, are you a comedian?"

She very positively surprised me, I really appreciated her comment and it made me like her right away, after that we started talking and I explained to her more about my job as a writer and motivational speaker.

That was a great example of both a cold read, so a blind guess on someone based off their actions or something they said, followed by a compliment.

You can make guesses about what they do, where they come from, what hobbies they have... and so on...

And believe me, it's far better than just asking questions as if it was an interview. Such as "So what is your job?" or "What do you do in your free time?"

There's no comparison.

It can really be anything, like, "Wow, you've such good taste in clothing, I bet you're a stylist.", "You are so convincing, you must be a great seller.".

If you guess correctly, they'll be even happier, they'll laugh and wonder how you knew. That means more bonus points for you.

But if you don't, it's okay, you will positively surprise the person you're talking to and make them like you right away.

It's a great method to get rid of the interview vibe, giving the conversation a fun pace. You make a guess, compliment them and as a consequence they will start telling you what they actually do or where they come from etc etc.

In addition, it is very likely that they will be much more involved in the conversation and they will show much more engagement and appreciation towards you.

CHAPTER 7:
THE AVALANCHE TECHNIQUE

The second method to progress after engaging in small talk is to create an avalanche of words, and in the midst of it, throw in a good question. Creating an avalanche is definitely an appropriate move after giving a Cold-Read.

The goal here is to ask a good question, it doesn't matter how simple, to put the other person in a position where they'll want to talk a lot.

This will make the other person feel really involved in the conversation, and it will ensure that you avoid getting those one-word answers you get when the other person is not really interested in the conversation.

So, the other person will be so excited about the question you asked them that they'll answer with a cascade of words.

There are two ways to achieve this reaction, that will work even better if combined together:

First of all you have avoid any question you can answer to with a yes or a no or that has no possible follow up whatsoever.

For example "For how long have you lived here?"

That's a question that's both trivial and that can end a conversation right then and there.

Most of the time people can just reply "10 months", "1 year" or other other answers along those lines.

Remember that you have to emotionally engage them by getting their feelings involved in order to create interest in the conversation.

"What do you like to do for fun? or "Why did you move here?" are both much more open questions that leave room for much longer answers, as well as make the other person talk about their own feelings.

The second key point is to ask them a question they are unconsciously waiting for and therefore they will want to answer, because it's about a topic they like.

It is very common among people to ask, for example, "Hey how's work?" This is a classic question that will generate a one word answer "good / bad / fine" and that will be the end of the exchange.

But if you get their feelings involved too, their answers will change drastically: "Hey, what's cool at work these days?" (this will push them towards talking about something they like or dislike about their job, a project or a co worker or who knows what else) or "hey, how are you spending your free time lately, what do you do for fun?" or even "Is anything exciting happening in your life right now?"

In addition to creating a positive atmosphere, there will be a better connection between the two of you and the person you are talking to will feel much more involved in the conversation.

CHAPTER 8:
THE GUESSING GAME

The third method for the most effective small talk is to play a guessing game.

The premise is to avoid doing this all the time, so not after every sentence, but first let's see what it actually consists of:

If you realize that you are about to ask one of those trivial routine questions such as "Where are you from?", you can turn it into a guessing game right away by saying something like. "Wait, wait, give me a couple of hints and let me see if I can guess."

They will now have to give you two hints and by thinking about those tips they will already be more involved in the conversation, plus they will appreciate the fact that you are trying to make the conversation more fun.

So, while you're guessing, you will also find yourselves joking and laughing.

Finding out where they are from will be a lot more fun this way.

It is a very useful method in most social situations and in various contexts such as bars, clubs, or any closed place really. Go for it whenever you think it is appropriate (use your common sense) it's a fun and refreshing way to ask instead of using the classic routine questions that feel so much like an interrogation of the FBI.

It's also much better than having the conversation go on and on about traffic, the weather, or other monotone subjects.

Let's face it, people always end up talking about that and it's boring.

45

CHAPTER 9:
GIVE ME YOUR ADVICE

The fourth and last method for successful small talk is to ask the person in front of you for an opinion on a topic you're interested in.

You will not necessarily have to keep talking about this topic but they will appreciate you asking for an opinion or advice and listening to them.

This will show them that you give importance and value to what they tell you or what they think.

This is all about asking a simple question about what you honestly think is interesting, and it's really nothing more than saying "Hey, I have a quick question for you, what do you think about...this or that?"

Unlike the second method in which we ask a question that you think could be interesting for them, here we ask a question about a topic of interest for us, based on what we like.

You can also play a little bit with them, for example, by asking a girl at the bar a question like: "Hey, which shirt do you like better, mine or his?" (pointing at some other random person at the bar) and after their answer playfully say: "Ah come on you're just saying that because you like him more than me, it's not the shirt."

This is guaranteed to create a fun and relaxed atmosphere.

If you want to keep the conversation more serious and discover something about the other person's way of thinking, say for example that they are married or divorced, you can ask something along the lines of "Hey, I've been together with my fiance for a while now and I've never been married, in your opinion, what makes a long-term relationship work?"

They will be excited to answer whether they have a successful marriage behind them or not, because people always have a tendency of giving tips to avoid mistakes they made themselves.

In this way you will be able to get an idea of the person's way of thinking, as well as make that person open up to you and it's much better than the usual trivial questions like "how's work going" or "what are you doing" etc.

CONCLUSION

Breaking the ice and approaching someone new is demonized and looked at as an insurmountable problem to solve.

In reality it is nothing like that and it should come as natural as possible.

Fixing your habits and improving your technique using the methods I illustrated in this book will do wonders.

Get back in action and never feel awkward again.

Try out these tricks and improve your social skills!

Best of luck see you in the next book.

ACKNOWLEDGEMENTS

The purpose of this book is to make your life better by improving your conversational skills and help you finally get rid of social awkwardness.

We want to thank you for taking action by reading this book and we hope that you keep on using these simple and efficient methods in order to reach your goal. If you found this helpful, we hope that you can spread the word to everyone around you who struggles with the same problems in order to help them.

We also want to thank all of the members of our publishing team for making this possible.

A special thanks goes also to all of the researchers who study this matter every day at the cost of their own sleep to help us improve our life.

Thank you all.